The Ultimate 21 Day

Sugar Detox Guide for Beginners

Lose Weight Quickly, Achieve Optimal Health, Feel Energized and Eliminate Sugar Cravings Naturally

Emma Rose

Table of Contents

Introduction

I want to thank you and congratulate you for purchasing this book!

This book contains proven steps and strategies on how to detoxify your body and kick Sugar Addiction in the butt within 21 days.

Because of the way food is processed nowadays, most people don't know that almost everything they eat has lots of sugar in it. And with sugar being discovered as the real cause of obesity, heart disease and other illnesses, this is a very bad thing.

Understand Sugar Addiction, its symptoms and the detrimental health effects it has. Know exactly what sugar does to your brain and body. And most importantly, know how exactly you can kick your sugar addiction goodbye!

All my life I've had a sweet tooth. I would even go as far as to say that I had a sugar addiction! Over the last few years my sugar addiction got worse: I had dessert multiple times a day and every day (I guess being a Foods teacher didn't help much). I would joke with people by telling them that I had my servings of vegetables for the day in chocolate...except, I still didn't have the vegetables. It got pretty bad. I knew I hated eating that much dessert but I couldn't stop. I would eat one Ferrero Rocher and then go back for another. As I walked back to the treats, I would pass the mirror and think to myself, "I don't need to have this chocolate. But, ah, what the heck, I don't care." In the end, I'd have about 6 Ferrero Rocher in addition to the other treats I had earlier that day.

Finally, I had to take the huge tray of Ferrero Rocher to school to give to my students on Valentine's Day. There was no way I could eat the other 30 myself. Eating all this sugar caused a huge war within me. I knew that my extreme sugar eating was unhealthy for me but I didn't want to stop. I loved it too much. As a result, I wrestled between the ideal of where I wanted to be and the reality of where I was. I knew I had the discipline to say no to other things, so why couldn't I say no to chocolate?

I eventually came to the point where I was starting to get fed up with not feeling well. I had a lot of chronic pain in my neck and I was constantly tired. I knew that sugar was irritating the problem and causing inflammation in my body. At was starting to reach the breaking point. Ultimately, I chose to go off of sugar for at least three weeks to break the habit I had created for myself. It was seriously a miracle to stay consistent with my goal because I really didn't want to give up my favorite desserts.

I encourage you to make that switch to healthier and happier lifestyle. Cutting out all the processed foods and going back to the basics really does clear up the body and help it function better. I've seen the changes in my own life as hard as it's been to make those changes. You, too, can make the changes necessary and still have your sweets along the way!

Thanks again for purchasing this book, I hope you enjoy it!

Please take some time to stop by and LIKE our Facebook page:

https://www.facebook.com/joypublishing

With gratitude, *Emma Rose*

Chapter 1

The Problem with Too Much Sugar...

For years, nutritionist have pinned all the caution warning on fats and other additives found in everyone's diets. But the real cause of all the obesity and other complications have been uncovered from the role it plays to weaken your diet and your body.

- *Sugar has no essential nutrients and spells trouble for your teeth.*

  A lot of sugar additives have high levels of calories with literally no essential nutrients, which is why they are called the Empty Calories. When it is said that there are no essential nutrients, it means no proteins, fats, vitamins or minerals, all that is in sugar is just pure energy. If the amount of sugar in your calorie intake goes up to 10 or 20 percent, you'll start having problems in nutrient deficiencies and more.

  Also, being a substance of easily convertible energy, it means that it is not only your body that gets a boost, so does the bad bacteria in your mouth. That could be a major disaster for your teeth. It feeds the bacteria so they multiply faster, harming your mouth (and body) faster.

- *Fructose can overload your liver.*

Sugar is broken down into two simple sugar compounds before it enters the bloodstream. These are fructose and glucose. Glucose can be found in every living cell in all organisms. If you don't consume enough of it from your foods, your body would provide it for you. Now the problematic one is fructose. It is not naturally occurring in your body so you can only get it through your diet. Your body does not really need fructose in order to function properly, but it does taste good.

Fructose is not inherently bad because we do get it from eating fruits, but the only organ that can metabolize it properly is the liver, and it stores the processed fructose as glycogen until your body needs it. Now, if the liver is already full of glycogen, it will transform the rest of the fructose (if you keep on digesting too much) into fat. And this can turn into a fatty-liver problem.

This is usually not a problem who are physically active. Healthy, active people metabolize their fructose faster before it can become a burden to their bodies. This is compared to people who have a sedentary lifestyle who ingest the same high-calorie, high-sugar diet.

- *Sugar can cause insulin resistance that can drive towards diabetes.*

We know that insulin helps the cells focus on burning glucose instead of fat when blood sugar enters these cells. Insulin resistance is caused by the insulin hormone stopping from working properly. Too much glucose in the blood is very toxic and causes the complications of diabetes, like going blind.

4

When the cells become resistant to insulin, the glucose stacks up in them and contributes to the onset of diseases. These may include obesity, metabolic syndrome, cardiovascular diseases and most commonly, diabetes (type II). Large amounts of sugar consumed have always been associated with insulin resistance.

- *Sugar has fat-promoting effects.*

Different food types have different effects on the brain and hormones, particularly those that deal with controlling the appetite. Glucose and fructose have opposite effects on the satiation of hunger.

In a certain medical study, those who drank fructose-sweetened beverages actually become hungrier while those sweetened with glucose got lowered levels of the hunger hormone, Ghrelin. Sugar can provide energy, but it cannot remove hunger, thus this contributes to an increase in calorie intake.

- *Sugar is highly addictive.*

Sugar causes massive releases of dopamine in the brain. This is like your brain rewarding the body for something it likes. Because of this, people susceptible to addiction become hooked to sugary foods as well as junk foods.

The problem in the saying "Everything in Moderation" is it does not work for people addicted to sugar. The only thing that will help with this true addiction is to completely remove sugars from your diet.

- *It's the sugar and not the fat that raises the cholesterol and contributes to heart disease.*

The world has always blamed saturated fats for heart diseases, which by the way, is the leading cause of death in the world. But, newer studies show that it is not fat but fructose that causes harm to the body's metabolism and thus contribute to diseases. That does not mean that fructose is inherently bad, only that the massive doses of fructose takes a toll on the body over time. After all, fructose is used in just about everything nowadays, especially sweetened beverages and processed food.

It has been proven that stacking up sugar in the blood and cells can raise the small, dense LDL and oxidized LDL triglycerides (also known as very bad stuff!) within mere weeks. And at the same time, the built up fructose also raise blood sugar, insulin levels and abdominal obesity. And this all spell risks for heart diseases.

Chapter 2

How Do You Know You're Addicted to Sugar?

Addiction to sugar is associated to a persistent imbalance in the blood sugar, letting the body show signs and symptoms for the condition. Here are a few observed behavioral and physiological signs that you've become addicted to sugar:

- You have a craving for bread products, sugary beverages, or sweets. This is the most common and easily discernible symptom, so keep watch.

- You have what they call the food coma. It is the feeling of drowsiness and fatigue after a heavy meal. It has always been attributed to eating too much, but now we know that this is the body trying to deal with the sugar influx.

- When you miss a meal, you get a feeling of lightheadedness. Sometimes, you might even feel faint and dizzy, with the accompanying sense of irritation because of bright lights (or even just regular light). If your body gets used to a high energy, high calorie intake every time, missing a meal can make your body go into withdrawal.

- When, after you eat some sweets you get a craving for more. Actually, you feel the craving more once you've eaten the sweets. This is because the fructose in the sugar, by encouraging production of ghrelin, increases the feeling of hunger. This makes for a good appetizer and a bad snack.

- You have become dependent on caffeine to get your body started. You keep looking for coffee and sodas in order to stay awake and keep going.

- You have hard time losing weight; more so than average people. This is not because of your genes and definitely not from being too fat. This is your body being too busy dealing with all that sugar to actually start burning fat.

Usually, these can be alleviated or even completely removed by balancing your blood sugar. Here are the tried and tested methods to do just that:

- Eat more proteins. Protein promotes muscle-building which can help to metabolize your excess fats. For this, you have to ensure that you are digesting them properly. You can check this by monitoring the levels of your stomach acids.

- Eliminate sugar and carbohydrates from your diet. They are good for instant energy but bad for your sugar addiction. Eating regular, healthy meals regularly should be sufficient for your energy needs.

- Eat more good fats, complex carbohydrates, fiber and essential nutrients. A craving for sugar can come from your body not getting enough nutrients. Fiber-rich foods are also great for detoxifying your body not only from the build-up of sugar, but also from fats and other toxins.

- Detoxify your body from sugar!

  It may prove to be a challenge at first, but doing the detox will definitely fix your blood sugar imbalance. And it will set up the stage for an opportunity to fix all other flaws in your diet.

It is reported that sugar addiction is even worse than other kinds of addiction. You might find that it is more difficult to get over, since there is sugar in almost everything you eat and drink, but once you have decided, and you successfully keep at it for these three weeks, you'll see results that you will be proud of.

Chapter 3

Why? How Do You Get Addicted?

It is estimated that sugar is around eight times more addictive than cocaine. Most people would have you think that sugar addiction is just a psychological eating disorder, or that it is just caused by your emotional state. That is not the case. It is a biological addiction, a disorder of the hormones and an error in the chemical balance in your body that causes cravings for sugars and carbohydrates. This will lead to uncontrollable binge eating. There has been a recent study showing that a high-sugar drink has the same addictive effect to the brain as a food-product spiked with cocaine or even morphine.

Most people would not notice that they have a full-blown sugar addiction. This is because they don't know that sugar is in everything that they eat. There was even an event where nutritionists requested food manufacturers to decrease the amount of sugar incorporated into their processed food by 30% to stop an incoming wave of diseases. Nobody reacted to the announcement because the idea was deemed absurd. What? There is sugar in a can of tomato soup? Actually, there is at least four teaspoons of sugar in each serving of that stuff.

When digesting sugar, your brain releases a kind of hormone that gives a wave of good feeling. And at the same time, that feeling activates the addiction center in the brain. Your body, liking the reaction from the stuff, will make you want more and more of it. Since sugar can be found in most food items available, you'll end up overeating, risking ingesting too much of both sugar and carbohydrates than what can be good for your body.

By developing a habit of having a constant high level of sugar in your blood, your body slowly gets used to this diet. Once you miss a meal or when you try to lower your blood sugar, your body then rejects the change. This is what happens when you experience "sugar withdrawal". Many would just use this excuse to eat more sugary sweets. But you have to see that it will only feel horrible at first. Slowly getting your diet back on the right track is worth the trouble.

Chapter 4

How Do Detox Works? Why Detox?

The detoxification works by over-correcting your body's sugar balance. This is done by completely removing sugars from your diet for a period of time to clear out any of the excess sugars before letting you return to your regular (not the sugary-regular, just regular) diet. This process can make you experience some effect that people call "Sugar Withdrawal Syndrome" that may last from a few days to a week. Mostly, it would be better to just muster up all your will power to get over these symptoms, since it will fade as you go along with the detox program. For those experiencing especially serious withdrawal symptoms, physical activity and drinking a lot of water every day will help a lot to ease the conditions. This will also include drinking water when you do feel the huge waves of food/sugar cravings that will attack you through the entire process.

So if the withdrawal can get unpleasant, why detox? Firstly, feeling worse about it actually means you are really getting better and that your body is getting rid of the built up sugar in your blood. Most of all, there are more benefits to sugar detox than just decreasing or removing your excessive craving for sweets. Some of these pluses are:

- You will begin to lose fat faster and easier. You might even find that your body's fat has gone down during the detox.

- You will feel less bloated. It is a feeling attributed to the time during or after a meal. Sugar imbalance also gives the bloated feeling that can persist throughout the day.

- Your tastes will return to normal. That would mean that healthier food will taste better since your sense is not tuned to preferring sweetness anymore. It is like removing your taste buds' bias towards sweet things. You'll be able to enjoy different kinds of food more.

- Your skin will appear clearer. Sugary diets zap out the collagen in your skin, making your complexion look blotchy and pallid. After detox, since you've lessened the sugar and increased water intake, you'll find that your skin has become better-looking than ever.

- You'll have more control over your hunger. After the detox process, you will see that you no longer have random attacks of cravings for sugar, or other food, for that matter.

- You'll have more energy and you'll feel it consistently throughout your day. There will be no more noon times after lunch spent being drowsy.

- You will have a more regular bowel movement. This is seen in detox diets that focus on removing excess sugar and carbs, promoting fiber and other essential nutrients in the process.

- Your attitude might improve, with less depressed moments and a general elevation of mood. Although this mostly comes from the knowledge that you are doing what is good for your body.

- You will definitely lower your body cholesterol; in fact, it would be great to combine this sugar detox program with physical exercise.

- You'll sleep better. A healthy diet usually helps create better sleeping habits.

Other than these physical and behavioral improvements, this sugar detox will also let you have a happier and healthier outlook on life that will help you set up the stage for creating the lifestyle that you have always wanted. Create a goal of making a lifestyle that will let you live longer, healthier, and happier!

Chapter 5

How to Start Detox?

There are basically three things you need to do during the sugar detox period. There are more to it like good exercise and removing other unhealthy diets as well. But for now these are the things you have to focus on:

1. You have to avoid eating or drinking all sugar and simple carbohydrates from your diet for 21 days, uninterrupted. There is a very long list of things you cannot eat compared to the much shorter one of recommended food. You must follow these at all times.

2. You have to watch what you eat for those three weeks. It would be recommended to keep a food journal for this task. Doing so will make it easier for you to watch out what you eat and you'll find it easier to control eating impulses. It can even encourage you to continue the food journal even after the detox period. You might also want to include a computation of your total calorie intake for each entry.

3. If you missed a day of detoxification or if you slip up and eat something you're not supposed to even just once (eating or drinking something with sugar or simple carbs), you'll have to start from zero. This will motivate you to try hurdling through the 21 days without returning to day one.

Before you do start the sugar detox process, you have to consider some of these things in your mind. But, just a warning: you have to hold steadfast. Remember what they say about beauty and health, "no pain, no gain". Not that you'll be in pain, for the most part. Here are some of the things you need to think about:

- *21 Days can feel like an eternity.*

    You may have chosen this detox plan on a whim. Maybe you just saw it in a forum or you heard someone who did well with it. Well, you'll see 21 days solidly spent on this detox is no walk in the park. It's going to be like crawling through briars in the middle of a thunderstorm. You have to keep your determination steadfast and just don't be discouraged because it will definitely prove to be a challenge. The rewards will all be worth it in the end, that's for sure.

- *You'll have to stick to it honestly.*

    Finishing your 21-day sugar detox within less than 21 days will be the easiest way to relapse into our sugar addiction. Cutting your diet plan this way will ensure the return of your problematic habit, probably more strongly than before. It is a carefully-made program that will ensure ridding both your body and your mind of the uncontrollable craving for sugar. So, just because you feel a little better after a week or two, you cannot just cut the detox process that short. It is set at 21 days for a reason.

    Absolutely don't cheat, shortcut or mess it up. If you did, even by the tiniest little bit, restart and do it properly for three weeks.

- *A one-time 3-week detox may not be enough.*

If you think a single three-week detox will work for you, don't be too sure. A lifetime worth of sugar addiction can take quite a few passes of this detox process to completely clear out. Advice: keep at it until you've been completely "cured" of the built up sugar over all those years. But do remember to take a break. Say after three weeks of uninterrupted detox, return to a normal (albeit a healthier) diet and then restart after some time following through the three weeks again.

- *It is not a lifestyle changing plan.*

It is just the tip of the ice berg, so to say. You have to decide what lifestyle you would be following after your detox. That is because you will definitely have to leave the high-carb, high-sugar lifestyle you've had before, so take a note of this. You can even use this opportunity to fix more than just your diet in your lifestyle. After all, it will be easier for you to change some of your unhealthy habits when you don't have those persistent cravings anymore. But note that this will just be a start if you want a complete lifestyle change.

- *It is adjustable to fit different individuals.*

Definitely better than most of the unchangeable diet programs, sugar detox can take form on different levels or intensity to suit your sugar use. There are some designed for those who have flat-out sugar addiction. While there is also some plans that is preferred by the ones who don't consume that much sugar, there are those that are made for slow-starters. Either that or it is because they feel that the higher level detox programs are too much. Being a bit uncomfortable with the designed plan is normal; you are trying to change your habits after all. But you should know that too much discomfort is detrimental to your progress. So, choose a detox plan that will suit your requirements.

- *The detox process pushes all the bad things out. It will let you feel in full what all that sugar was doing to your body.*

You will definitely feel the effects of withdrawal. The worst of the effects of that built up sugar in your body will certainly show themselves during the process. Remember to keep your determination to help you overcome these things and the experiences that will obstruct the path of your detoxification in the first few days.

Your nutritionist or physician can suggest further additions to this diet as well as other things you can do to make it more effective. They can give helpful advice such as the kind of physical activity you can maintain during the detox period. If you didn't want to consult with a doctor, you can find many references on the subject. There are many discussions about tried and tested diet plans in books, articles and blogs online.

Chapter 6

Some Sugar-free Recipes

Here are some of the food products you would want to have in your diet during the sugar detox program:

- Herbs

- Vegetables (except potatoes)

- Beans

- Avocado

- Carrots

- Coconut Oil

- Eggs

- Fish

- Meat

- Nuts

- Olive Oil

- Seed-foods

- Tomatoes

- Citrus Fruits (not the sweet citrus ones though)

- Unsweetened chocolate (Dark and black chocolates are actually good for you. Even if they're quite bitter, they can substitute desserts. It is an acquired taste after all so they might take a little getting used to.)

And the stuff you need to avoid:

- Alcohol

- Flour and flour-based products

- Fried food

- Fruit juices

- Artificial sweeteners (they're worse than sugar, promise!)

- fruits

- Bread products

- Corn syrup (start checking labels, this stuff is in many things)

- Candy

- honey

- Cereal

- Maple syrup

- Cheese

- Potatoes (yes, even fries)

- Dairy products

- oatmeal

- Cream sauces

- Sugar

- Soy

- Tortillas and other corn-based crackers

- White rice

- Trans-fat (these should be in the label, look them up)

- Yogurt (even the non-fat, unsweetened ones!)

- Pasta (all of them)

- Pizza

Meatballs in Tomato Sauce

Ingredients:

- ¼ cup Parmesan cheese
- 2 lightly beaten eggs
- 1/3 cup whole wheat bread crumbs
- 12 oz. or 3 pieces sausages removed from casings
- 1 lb. ground beef (choose one with less fat)
- 1 tsp. minced garlic
- Salt
- Pepper
- Parmesan cheese for garnish

Sauce:
- 1 tbsp. minced garlic
- 2 cans tomatoes, diced and pureed
- 1 tsp. dried oregano
- 2 tsp. dried basil
- salt

Procedure:

1. Preheat the oven to 425° F. Remove the sausages and ground beef from the cold. Squeeze the sausage meat from their casings and bring both meats to room temperature.

2. Put the bread crumbs in a bowl and add 1/3 cup of hot water. Let the crumbs absorb the water before adding the garlic, salt, pepper, grated Parmesan cheese and the eggs. After mixing them well, add the meats and use your hands to combine them.

3. Prepare the pan or dish with oil or nonstick spray. Round up meatballs with your hands, using a spoon to measure out the meat. Arrange them so they'll have space between each meatball.

4. Puree the tomatoes. After putting it in a bowl, add in the salt, herbs and garlic. Pour this sauce over the meatballs. Sprinkle the remaining cheese over them. Bake them until the sauce and the cheese is bubbling. That would take just over half an hour.

Serve it hot with more Parmesan sprinkled on the meatballs.

This recipe makes about 6 servings.

Chicken Nuggets with Almonds

Ingredients:

- 2 tbsp. olive oil
- 1 tsp. paprika
- ½ cup almond flour or almond meal
- ½ tsp. chicken seasoning
- 2 skinless chicken breasts, boneless

Procedure:

1. Preheat oven to 400° F. Prepare the pan and baking sheet with the olive oil.

2. Remove all tendons and visible fat from the chicken then cut it into nuggets (each breast piece should make about 5 pieces). Make sure they are all of the same thickness, using a kitchen mallet to even out differences.

3. Combine the rest of the ingredients in a bowl and mix well. Dip each nugget into this mixture, making sure it coats the chicken evenly. Line them up into the pan with the baking sheet.

4. Cook for around 10 minutes, until the side touching the pan is slightly browned. The nuggets become too hard and chewy when overcooked so don't overdo it. Once one side is cooked, turn the nuggets and then cook for another 10 minutes.

5. Serve hot with your favorite chicken nugget dip.

This recipe makes about 2 servings.

Muffin Pan Meal

Ingredients:

- 6 eggs
- 8 ½ oz. muffin mix (or corn bread)
- Salt
- Pepper
- 15 oz. corned beef

Procedure:

1. Grease the 12-cup muffin pan. Divide the corned beef into six of these cups. Press them down, so that it sticks to the bottom and comes up at the sides to form shells.

2. Break an egg into each shell and season with some salt and pepper.

3. Prepare muffin mix according to the instructions on the packaging. Spoon the muffin batter into the remaining 6 cups.

4. Bake at 400° F for up to 20 minutes or just when the muffins are golden brown.

5. Put the cooked egg and shell onto the muffins as toppings. Serve immediately. They could also be reheated by putting them through the microwave for a few seconds on mid-level heat.

This recipe makes 4 - 6 servings.

Chicken Skillet

Ingredients:

- 3 tbsp. olive oil
- ½ chopped green pepper
- 1 chopped onion
- 4 crushed garlic cloves
- 1 ½ lbs. boneless chicken
- Salt
- Pepper

Procedure:

1. Slice the chicken to your desired serving pieces.

2. Heat the oil in the skillet and cook the chicken until they are nearly done.

3. Add the garlic, onion and the green pepper, sauté them with the chicken.

4. You know you are finished cooking when the chicken is slightly browned and the onion has become soft.

5. After that, you can add some choice vegetables and sauté until cooked to your liking.

6. Season with salt and pepper.

Beef Barbecue Sandwiches and Burritos

Ingredients:

- Hamburger buns
- 1 packet taco seasoning
- Flour tortillas with your favorite toppings
- 1 bottle of barbecue sauce
- 5 lbs. roast beef

Procedure:

1. Shred well-cooked roast meat with a fork. Reserve half of the meat for the sandwiches. Drain any liquid left in the pot with the meat. Put the taco seasoning and stir in two cups of water with the remaining half of the meat. Cook until heated through.

2. Serve on tortillas.

3. Take the other half and stir in the barbecue sauce. Heat mixture in the microwave (or on a stove top).

4. Serve on buns.

This recipe makes about 4 servings.

Onion Rings

Ingredients:

- 2 onions, choose the white ones
- ½ red pepper powder or chili powder
- 1 tsp. ground black pepper
- Salt
- 250 ml beer
- 1 ¾ cup flour
- ¼ cup corn meal

Procedure:

1. Mix the flour and corn meal, stirring in the red and black pepper, salt and beer. Make sure all the ingredients are mixed evenly. Afterwards, cover it and let it sit for an hour.

2. In a pan, heat about 5 cm-high peanut or olive oil until it is around 370° F.

3. On a plate filled with a mound of flour, toss 5 or 6 pieces of onion rings, and then dip it in your prepared batter. Drop them one at a time into the oil.

4. Cook the rings for a few minutes until they are sufficiently browned on both sides. Drain off all oil with paper towels or by putting them on a wire rack. Salt the rings and serve hot.

This recipe makes 4-6 servings.

Eggplant Sticks

Ingredients:

- ½ cup beaten eggs
- ¾ tsp. garlic and salt powder
- 1 cup spaghetti sauce or tomato sauce of your choice
- 1 eggplant (1 ¼ lbs.)
- Seasoning of your choice

Procedure:

1. Cut eggplant into snack-sized sticks.

2. In a long bowl or on a dish, combine the garlic and salt powder, with your choice seasoning. Dip each eggplant stick into the beaten eggs then coat it in the powder mixture. Arrange them on a baking sheet.

3. Spray the laid out sticks with cooking spray. Broil the sticks for 3 minutes. Remove the baking sheet from the oven afterwards.

4. Turn the sticks and spritz them again with the cooking spray. Cook for another 2 minutes or when they are browned to your liking.

5. Serve hot. Prepare the tomato sauce as your dip.

This recipe makes about 8 servings.

Sausage Snacks

Ingredients:

- 12 oz. spicy pork sausages, ground
- 12 oz. pork sausages, ground
- Ham slices
- Scrambled eggs, fried
- mayonnaise

Procedure:

1. Preheat your broiler.

2. Mix and cook the ground pork sausage and the spicy ground pork sausage in a well-oiled skillet. Brown the ground pork over medium high heat. Drain the sausage of any liquid.

3. Process the ground pork with the mayonnaise until they are incorporated well.

4. On each ham slice, place some of the ground pork mixture and some scrambled eggs. Roll them up and secure with a toothpick.

5. Broil the rolls for 3 to 5 minutes. Check it frequently, and finishing when they are sufficiently toasted.

This recipe makes about 5-6 servings.

Roasted Chickpeas

Ingredients:

- Olive oil or cooking spray
- Salt
- 1 tsp. chili powder
- 1 tsp. paprika
- 1 tsp. coriander
- 1 tsp. cumin
- 1 tsp. garlic powder
- 1 tsp. curry powder

Procedure:

1. Preheat oven to 375° F. Drain chickpeas and let them completely dry. You can pat dry with a paper towel.

2. Arrange them on a baking sheet, laying them on a single layer. Roast for around half an hour, shaking the pan every ten minutes. Just make sure they don't burn. You'll know they are done when they have turned golden brown with crunchy insides instead of moist.

3. Combine all the spices in a bowl, mixing them well. Remove the chickpeas from the oven when they are done and spray them with olive oil.

4. Toss the chickpeas with the spices while still hot.

5. They are preferably served hot. But you can also let them cool in room temperature and then place them in airtight Ziploc bags afterwards.

This recipe makes about 3 servings.

Conclusion

Thank you again for purchasing this book!

I hope this book was able to help you to have a less-sugary diet and have a more positive outlook to set you up for a good and healthy lifestyle.

The next step is to create a new lifestyle that will let you live healthier and happier.

In addition, please remember to check out our Facebook page in order to find other resources and upcoming promotions:

https://www.facebook.com/joypublishing

With sincere thanks,

Emma Rose

Preview Of "Paleo Desserts: Satisfy Your Sweet Tooth With Over 100 Quick and Easy Paleo Dessert Recipes and Paleo Baking Recipes"

Chapter 1

Brief History of Paleo Diet

The Sweet Effects

Why do you love sweet food? Why do you crave for more of that dessert so much? Your anatomy would tell you that sweet foods would cause the release of dopamine in the part of the brain that is associated with motivation and reward. Not only that, but studies show that sweets also produce an increased level of serotonin. Serotonin gives you that feeling of happiness and wellbeing. That's why it is better to give a box of chocolates when you want the person to be in a good mood.

Unfortunately, the quote you can't have your cake and eat it too applies here. The bad effects that sugar brings are common knowledge. The number one disease is diabetes. People are aware of diabetes and its complications. That is why even when you intensely crave for that delicious dessert, you try to control your urges and settle for nothing instead. Well, that is if your self-control is in good condition. More often than not, people would rather risk the medical condition and eat that sweet thing with all their heart.

I have had many slip ups in my own life. I went two months without chocolate...can you believe it? Then Easter came. I found that if I gave myself an inch, I would take a mile. Eating chocolate quickly got out of control. I rebelled because I was strict for so long. You may find yourself in the same situation and find it hard to balance the sugar cravings. Once the sugar cravings are there, your body craves more and then a vicious cycle begins.

Bonus Recipe:

Classic Chocolate-Strawberry Bars

This has many prehistoric ingredients but worth the effort.

Ingredients:
2 ¼ cups almond flour
½ cup coconut sugar
½ tsp baking powder
6 tbsp flaxseed meal
¼ tsp sea salt
2/3 cups arrowroot powder

6 tbsp coconut oil, melted
3 tbsp coconut milk
2 tsp vanilla extract

½ cup dark chocolate chips
½ cup fresh cut strawberries
1 tbsp fresh lemon juice

Handful chopped almonds (optional)

Procedure:

Preheat the oven to 350°F. Combine in a bowl 2 ¼ cups almond flour, ½ cup coconut sugar, ½ teaspoon baking powder, 6 tablespoons flaxseed meal, ¼ teaspoon sea salt and 2/3 cups arrowroot powder. In a separate bowl, whisk the following: 6 tablespoons melted coconut oil, 3 tablespoons coconut milk and 2 teaspoons vanilla extract. Mix together the wet and dry ingredients using a gloved hand. This will form soft dough. Take note not to over mix this.

Reserve ½ cup of dough to be used later. Place the remaining dough on an 8" x 8" baking pan lined with parchment paper. Top with ½ cup dark chocolate chips. Cover the chips with fresh cut strawberries. Drizzle with 1 tablespoon fresh lemon juice and then drizzle with the extra dough plus an extra handful of almonds. Bake the dough for 20 minutes then lower the heat to 325°F and then bake for another 10 minutes. It should turn into a beautiful golden color crumble bar. Cut and serve.

Check out the rest of this book on Amazon.

Or go to: http://amzn.to/1lZNcVI

Check Out My Other Books

Below you'll find some of my other books also available on Amazon and Kindle. Search for these titles on the Amazon website to find them.

Paleo Free Diet Guide for Beginners: Over 50 Paleo Free Recipes for Optimal Health & Fast Weight Loss

Paleo Desserts: Satisfy Your Sweet Tooth With Over 100 Quick & Easy Paleo Dessert Recipes & Paleo Baking Recipes

Raw Food Diet Guide: Lose Weight Quickly, Achieve Optimal Health & Feel Energized with the Raw Food Diet & Raw Food Recipes

Clean Eating Guide: Lose Weight Quickly, Achieve Optimal Health & Feel Energized with Clean Eating For Busy Families & Clean Eating Recipes

Alkaline Diet Guide: Lose Weight Quickly, Achieve Optimal Health & Feel Energized with the Alkaline Diet & Alkaline Recipes

Coconut Flour Recipes for Optimal Health & Quick Weight Loss: Gluten Free Recipes for Celiac Disease, Gluten Sensitivities & Paleo Free Diets

Almond Flour Recipes for Optimal Health & Quick Weight Loss: Gluten Free Recipes for Celiac Disease, Gluten Sensitivities & Paleo Free Diets

Wheat Free Diet for Beginners: Lose Weight Quickly, Achieve Optimal Health & Feel Energized with Gluten Free Recipes for Celiac Disease, Gluten Sensitivities & Paleo Free Diets

Detox Diet Guide: Lose Weight Quickly, Achieve Optimal Health & Feel Energized Through the 10 Day Detox

Sugar Detox Guide for Beginners: Lose Weight Quickly, Achieve Optimal Health, Feel Energized & Eliminate Sugar Cravings Naturally

Ketogenic Diet Guide for Beginners: How to Achieve Rapid Weight Loss, Optimal Health & Unstoppable Energy with Ketogenic Diet Recipes

Anti Inflammatory Diet for Beginners: Lose Weight Fast, Optimize Health, Slow Aging, Fight Inflammation, Conquer Pain & Increase Energy with the Anti Inflammation Diet Recipes

One Last Thing...

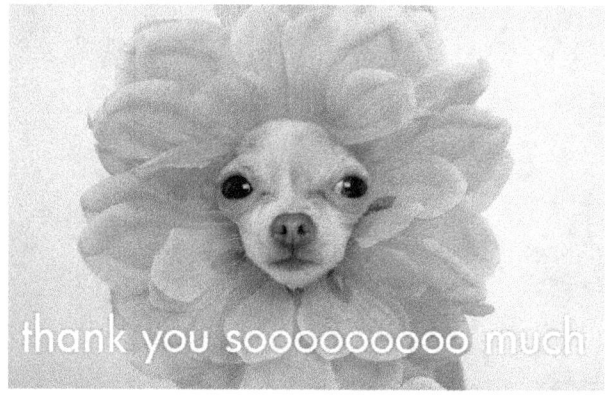

Source: Wikipedia

If you believe that this book is worth sharing, would you please take the time to let others know how it affected your life? If it turns out to make a difference in the lives of others, they will be forever grateful to you, as will I.